WEIGHT LOSS

HOW TO LOSE EXTRA WEIGHT

STEP BY STEP

1. 8 reasons why you should not lose weight

2. Obesity

3. Unexpected foods hinder weight loss

4. Slimming belt: is it effective in losing weight ?

5. Study: Eating While Walking Increases Weight

6. What is the difference between losing weight and losing fat ?

7. Staples at lunch for weight loss

8. A study says chewing gum saves weight

9. Basic tips and rules for controlling weight

10. 8 hormones that cause weight gain in women

11. Weight loss oils

12. The fastest way to lose extra weight

13. How to maintain weight after dieting

14. Genetic examination and genetic map to help with weight loss

1. 8 REASONS WHY YOU SHOULD NOT LOSE WEIGHT

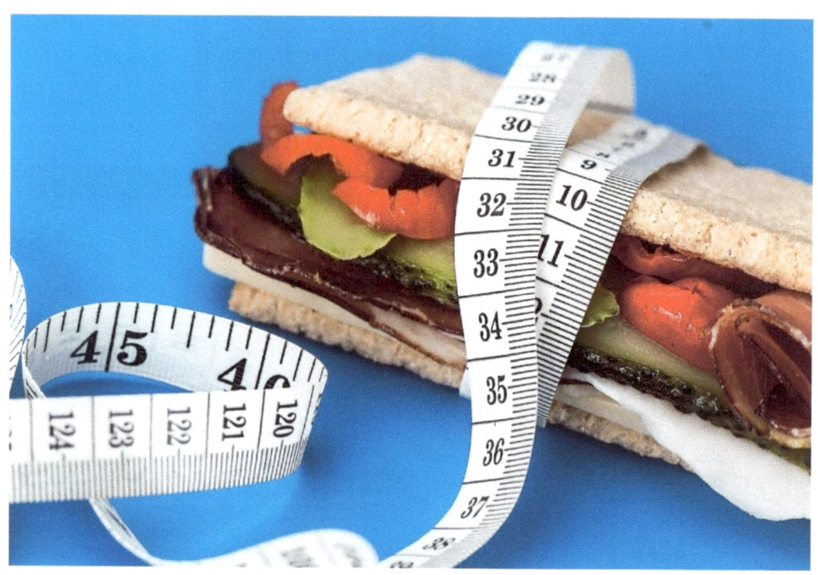

Have you ever substituted fries and soda for various diets, but are you continue to an equivalent weight? These are the foremost important reasons for not losing weight.

You'll think that eating small amounts of food will assist you reduce and provides you a slim figure. this will happen when people discuss the explanations for not losing weight before starting different weight loss diets. Here are the 8 most vital reasons to not lose weight:

• REASONS FOR NOT LOSING WEIGHT :

There are many possible reasons for not losing weight that a lot of might suffer from, and here we'll mention the foremost important reasons for not losing that weight:

• WATER :

Not drinking enough water during the day can put you in danger for obesity, as water makes up about 60% of your body and features a big effect on your weight, so drinking moderate amounts of water before meals helps. suppress appetite and reduce the amount of calories. .
This was a 12-week weight loss study that found people that drank half a liter of water half-hour before meals lost about 44% more weight compared to to people .

• DIETETIC FOODS :

Many diet foods contain abundant fat and hidden calories, and that they increase your sugar cravings and lower your energy levels, which results in weight gain over time.
Foods such as: oats, low-fat yogurt, and gluten-free foods often contain additives of sugar and fructose, which results in increased sugar within the body and its accumulation as fat within the hips and the abdomen.

Although soft drinks don't contain sugar, they are doing contain artificial sweeteners that your body cannot easily digest, which causes them to maneuver through the intestine, and thanks to glucose intolerance and hyperglycemia, the behavior of intestinal bacteria can change, turning these substances into fat, so one should choose diet products.After looking closely at his label, this is often one among the explanations he has not lost weight.

• DAILY MEALS :

Skipping meals can cause you to realize more weight rather than losing it. it's going to seem logical that eating less food while skipping a meal might assist you reduce , but skipping meals is usually counterproductive for several reasons, including:

The body's metabolism works best with regular meals because the body burns calories during the digestion process, but once you stop eating enough food, your metabolism rate slows down.

Once you don't eat enough food, your body reacts in reverse by preserving food as fat for energy.

For instance , skipping breakfast can cause you to hungrier around lunch and you'll overeat at that point .

• SLEEP :

Not getting enough sleep, this will be one more reason to extend weight, the sleep premium is abundant in the dark , it stimulates hunger hormones and increases appetite, resulting in weight gain over time, this which indicates that lack of sleep is one among the foremost important risk factors along side obesity, adults and youngsters that suffer from insufficient sleep have a 55% and 89% risk of affected by obesity, respectively.

To support your weight loss efforts, confirm you get 7-8 hours of sleep per day.

• PROTEINS :

Not eating enough protein can cause you to suffer from excess weight, and a high protein diet is sweet for weight loss because it reduces cravings for sugar and prevents excess fat from the build-up of fat sugar.
Where one study indicated that a high protein diet induces a sense of fullness and controls appetite, which helps in weight loss.

• MEDICINES :

The side effects of some medications could also be a explanation for your weight gain, as some prescribed drugs wont to treat depression, diabetes, heart attacks, migraines, and high vital sign can cause weight gain, so if you're trying to reduce while taking prescription medication, this might be one among the explanations why you're not losing weight. Additionally, some medications can increase your appetite and cause hunger pangs, and there also are people who hamper the metabolism or cause water retention, so if you notice your weight gain soon after taking the drug medication, don't stop it before seeing a doctor or getting an alternate .

• HYPOTHYROIDISM :

Hypothyroidism may be a disorder that affects the thyroid, which is liable for secreting fat-burning hormones, so when the body makes less of those hormones, your body finishes up burning fewer calories and storing them as fat. fats that accumulate after a period. of your time and cause a drastic increase in weight.

• FRUIT JUICES :

fruit crush is high in sugars and lacks fiber, protein, and healthy fats that cause you to feel more full. this will cause you to snack between main meals, increasing your daily calorie intake.

alittle orange can have around 45 calories, which is low and good for your body, but once you plan to make a cup of juice, you would possibly need 3 to 4 oranges, which can get you 180 calories in a couple of minutes.

2. OBESITY

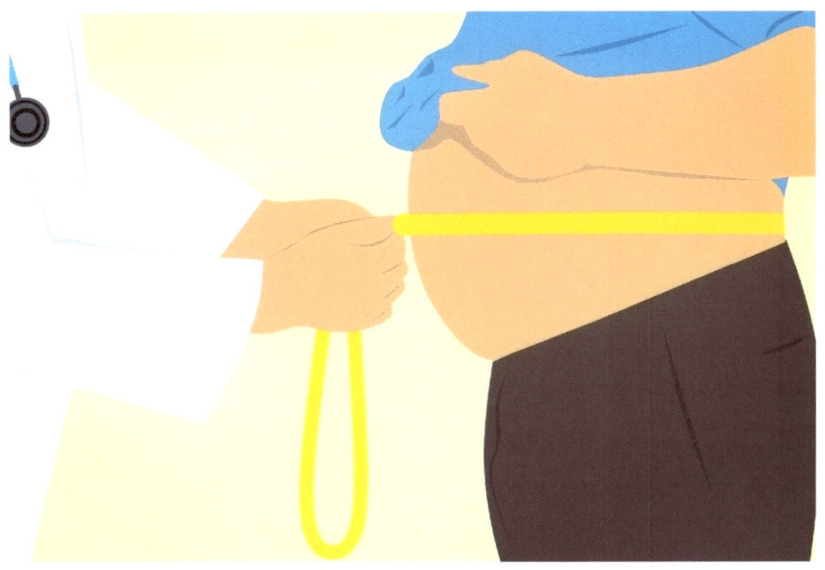

The definition of an obese person is a person who has excess fat tissue and has a body mass index (BMI) value of over 30. BMI is an indicator that measures weight compared to height. Excessive fatty tissue can have serious health consequences such as diabetes, high blood pressure and high levels of lipids in the blood.

The obesity is one of the most common medical conditions in Western society today, the most difficult in terms of the treatment of obesity and response. Relatively little progress has been made in treating obesity (with the exception of lifestyle changes), but much information has been collected regarding the medical consequences of obesity.

Until recently, obesity was related to a lazy (sitting) lifestyle and excessive calorie consumption. Today, however, it's known that these causes of obesity are important, but there also are different genetic factors that play a task within the onset of obesity.
As evidence, in adopted children we see a pattern of obesity that's almost like what we see in their birth parents, quite what we see in their adoptive parents. Research with identical twins has also shown that the effect of genetic factors on BMI is bigger than the influence of environmental factors thereon.
It's estimated that between 40% and 70% of obesity are often attributed to varied genetic factors, not environmental or lifestyle factors.

As research in mice has shown, the presence of 5 genes associated with appetite, these genes are those that cause obesity. These genes also are present in humans. one among the most genetic factors in obesity is that the hormone leptin.

Today, obesity is assumed to be a mixture of certain genes and not just the results of one defect during a gene. the rise in obesity in recent decades is especially thanks to environmental influences like lifestyle and eating habits.

• COMPLICATIONS OF OBESITY :

Obesity is related to higher rates of death and disease. There are an outsized number of diseases that are more common in people with obesity, high vital sign, type 2 diabetes, hyperlipidemia, arteria coronaria disease, degenerative joint disease and psychosocial disorders. It should be noted that patients with obesity often also suffer from metabolic syndrome (metabolic syndrome), which incorporates a minimum of three of the subsequent symptoms: girth of an outsized belly, high vital sign, high rate of fat within the blood, high level of sugar within the blood During fasting, low level of HDL (low level of excellent cholesterol).

Additionally , obesity is linked to the subsequent diseases: bowel, ovarian and carcinoma , embolism and hypercoagulability, diseases of the gastrointestinal system (gallbladder bag disease and heartburn) and various skin disorders.
Women who are obese during pregnancy have a better risk of developing complications as a results of childbirth and pregnancy.
Obese people suffer more from lung diseases and various endocrine disorders, like apnea and hormone secretion disorders.

• OBESITY DIAGNOSIS :

As mentioned earlier, obesity is defined as an more than adipose tissue.

Accurate measurement of body fat is complicated and requires professional evaluation. However, with an easy physical examination, the presence of excess fat are often easily detected. The Body Mass Index (BMI) provides a comparatively good estimate of the quantity of adipose tissue (in people with little muscle, like professional bodybuilders). BMI is calculated by dividing the load in kilograms by the square of the peak in meters.

Indication of BMI values:

18.5-24.9 - normal weight.

25-29.9- Overweight.

30-34.9- Obesity grade 1.

Obesity 35 to 39.9 grade 2.

Over 40 means obesity.

Upper obesity (central obesity), that is, the buildup of excess fat within the abdominal region and above the waist (abdominal circumference greater than 102 cm in men and greater than 88 cm in women), is of greater medical importance than lower obesity, that is, the buildup of excess fat within the buttocks and thighs.
People with higher obesity have a better risk of diabetes, stroke, disorder, and premature death than people with lower obesity.

• TREATMENT OF OBESITY :

Various dietary techniques are often followed, leading to weight loss and excess adipose tissue. Studies have shown that only 20% of patients are ready to process and lose 6 kg of their weight and maintain the new weight for 2 years.
The nutritional instructions for obese people are almost like those for normal people:

Increase the consumption of unprocessed foods that are given within the diet.

Limit your intake of fat, sugar, and alcohol.

• EAT FOODS HIGH IN FIBER :

Consistent with research, there was no significant and healthy preference for one method of treating obesity over another.

However, it's vital to teach patients about the treatment of obesity, the way to plan the daily menu early, and the way to record meals that are eaten. Behavioral education within the treatment of obesity is that the cornerstone of the way to reduce the right way.

Exercise is important for maintaining future weight loss and treating obesity. Physical activity results in a rise within the consumption of calories within the body.

It's important to worry and stress that exercise alone leads to slight weight loss. the most advantage of exercise is that it helps maintain weight loss over time.

Today, it's recommended to practice moderate to intense physical activity for one hour each day.

• MEDICAL TREATMENT OF OBESITY :

Only a few prescription obesity medications are approved and are recommended for weight loss. The drugs are recommended as a part of a comprehensive treatment program and not because the only method of treating weight loss and obesity.

• SURGERY :

People that are obese and have a BMI over 40 can have various stomach surgeries (balloon shortening, etc.) that cause weight loss.
But the decrease in weight, estimated at around 50% of the patient's initial weight, is amid side effects and high complications of the surgery, such as infection of the peritoneum, stones within the bile ducts, hypercoagulability and high nutritional disorders. with a deficiency of varied vitamins. Research also shows that around 40% of patients will experience complications from the surgery.

Conclusion :

Obesity is more and more common.
This phenomenon involves many injuries, within the quality of life and therefore the average age of an obese person.
Today there are many methods of treating obesity and weight loss, the essential principle on which these methods are based is to follow a healthy lifestyle, which incorporates exercise and diet. Healthy and balanced. In extreme cases, medication or surgery could also be used, but it's advisable to not come up with a situation that needs these procedures to treat obesity.

3. UNEXPECTED FOODS HINDER WEIGHT LOSS

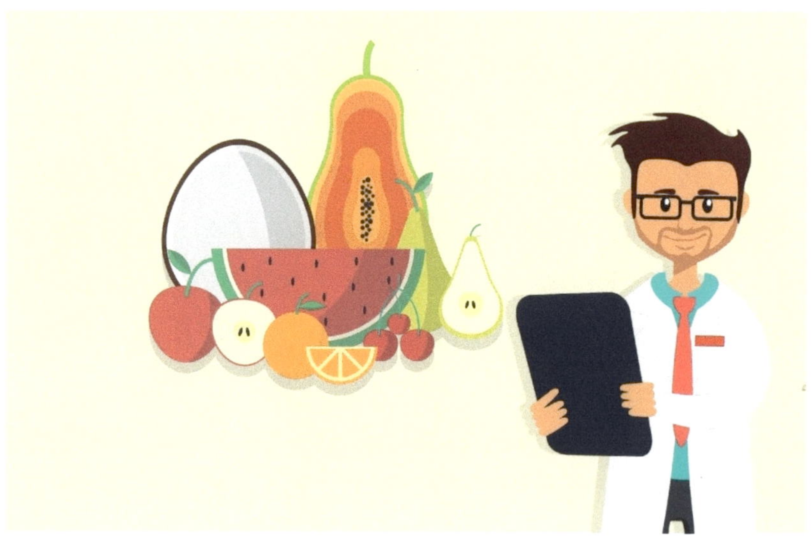

Are you trying to reduce but you can't? The foods you eat could also be the reason! determine the foremost important foods that hinder weight loss.

You would possibly be surprised to seek out that certain healthy foods that you simply want to eat all the time or foods known to be healthy are hampering all of your weight loss efforts.

Therefore, you would like to return your information about the foods that are right for you while dieting to maneuver within the right direction for weight loss.

• FAT-FREE DAIRY PRODUCTS :

Many avoid yogurt and whole or semi-skimmed milk and believe that skimmed milk is great for dieting and doesn't help with weight gain.
This is often because yogurt or skim milk can cause weight gain, because it's not as saturated as milk, and thus increases the sensation of hunger.
Also, some companies provide skimmed milk with sugar to sweeten it until the flavour is improved.
Skimmed milk provides the body with fewer nutrients than others, as milk is an important source of fat soluble vitamins, including vitamins A, D, E, and K, additionally to calcium and phosphorus.
These vitamins need fats to enter and absorb them into the body, and thus fat removal is difficult to soak up these vitamins.
Additionally, dairy products are generally acidic, whether fatty or fat free, and these acids contribute to the problem of losing weight.

• ALL TYPES OF FLOUR :

Many of us believe that whole wheat bread is that the best during a diet, and it's considered to be the healthiest type that helps with weight loss.

And while a limited intake of whole wheat could also be appropriate initially during the diet, continuing to eat wheat products (especially gluten) are often detrimental to weight loss because you will not feel full.

Whole wheat also causes the buildup of fat within the abdomen, and it also results in decreased energy levels within the body, and thus a scarcity of serious movement to reduce weight.

• PRODUCTS LABELED "LOW IN FAT" :

Dieters resort to buying "low fat" products, which is another trick some companies resort to as they replace taste with other things, often sugar or sodium.

Sugar is an acidic ingredient like dairy products, which inspires the body to stay the additional weight.

Also, foods that contain additional sodium and salt can cause bloating and cause you to feel heavier, and also contribute to weight gain.

• TOSSED SALAD :

Before eating a salad, you would like to form sure its ingredients, that it contains fresh vegetables which it's freed from any excess fats, oils, sauces or salts, and this is often what happens.

Often in ready-to-eat salads at restaurants.
Where restaurants store salads for long periods of time, which lose their nutritional value, and until they turn good, other items that hide the old taste, like cheese or toast, their are added.
A colourful salad with fresh, homemade vegetables is that the most beneficial and helps in weight loss.

• Dried fruits :

Some sorts of edible fruit contain amounts of hidden sugar and are therefore not suitable for those on a diet.
But that does not mean that each one dried fruits contain sugar, as there are healthy, sugar-free types, and this will be experienced by watching the ingredients listed on the package.
Your best bet is to eat fresh fruit, faraway from edible fruit, to form sure you're getting the complete advantage of its health benefits.
However, you ought to avoid the kinds of fruit that increase weight, like dates, mangoes, grapes, and much of fruits suitable for eating, like guava, oranges, and apples.

4. SLIMMING BELT : IS IT EFFECTIVE IN LOSING WEIGHT ?

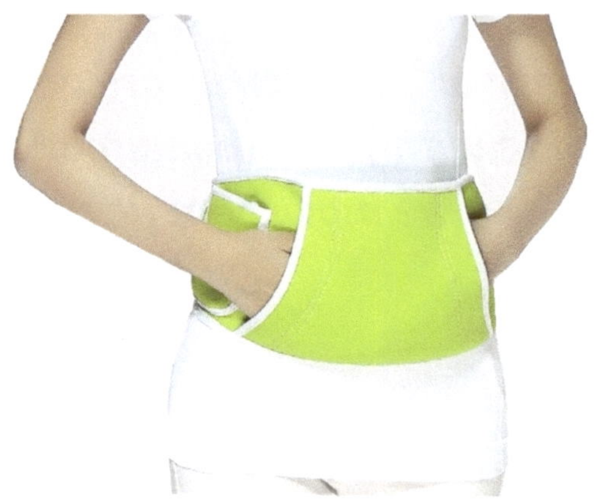

Recently it's become popular to use what's called the slimming belt for weight loss, but is it really an efficient method? How it works ? Are there any risks related to its use?

Many of us suffer from overweight, so overweight results in many problems like change in outward appearance, decrease in self-confidence.

• Appearance reducing self-confidence :

It also has many adverse health effects.
There are some ways to reduce, including diet and exercise.
But there are claims that modern methods like the slimming belt are effective in losing weight.

But before using the slimming belt, it's important to understand what the slimming belt is? How does it work to lose weight? Is it really useful ?

• what's the slimming belt ? :

The slimming belt is usually used for weight loss, and it's worn round the abdomen and lower back. The principle of operation of the slimming belt is straightforward.
It helps the body to sweat tons when wearing it, which helps burn calories, shrink stomach area, and reduce
There also are slimming belts that contain a vibration system to hurry up the calorie burning process.
The wearing time of the slimming belt varies counting on the merchandise and therefore the instructions mentioned, some products recommend wearing it for half-hour, and a few throughout the day.
But it's advisable to diet and exercise, because the belt alone isn't enough for weight loss.

• SLIMMING BELT MECHANISM :

The slimming belt acts to scale back weight because of the subsequent mechanisms :

INCREASED SWEATING :

Wearing a slimming belt increases an individual's perspiration, but what many of us do not know is that it causes an individual to lose water only his body only and no fat. If you wear a slimming belt during exercise, it increases sweating, but this is often not an honest thing because it's vital to stay the physical body hydrated during exercise. Excessive water loss during exercise impairs the power to perform exercise with high efficiency, and wearing a slimming belt doesn't necessarily mean that sweating is caused only by the stomach area.

SQUEEZE FAT CELLS :

Once you wear the slimming belt, it compresses the stomach and abdomen to seem smaller. But the purpose is that when you're taking off the slimming belt, the fat cells that have shrunk as a results of wearing it return to their original size, which suggests that you simply don't lose fat in the least by using the slimming belt. But you simply lose water.

THE PERSON'S POSITION :

If you suffer from poor posture while standing, wearing a slimming belt around your stomach and back helps improve posture and straighten your back. But wearing a slimming belt for an extended time prevents you from using the muscles in your back and abdomen, which weakens those muscles and worsens upright posture over time.
You will dispense with the rear belt and improve alignment by doing exercises that strengthen the rear muscles and therefore the front muscles.

SIDE EFFECTS OF THE SLIMMING BELT :

The utilization of the slimming belt could also be related to the looks of certain side effects :

SKIN PROBLEMS

Once you wear a slimming belt for long periods of your time, it causes skin sensitivity thanks to the heat and prolonged sweating.

DROUGHT

It's possible that dehydration is thanks to prolonged wear of the slimming belt, thanks to the loss of an outsized amount of water.
Here are the most signs of dehydration :

XEROSTOMIA.

INSOMNIA.

DECREASED URINE VOLUME.

A HEADACHE.

WE DRY THE SKIN.

DIZZINESS.

• INTERNAL ISSUES :

Slimming belt causing problems with wear and tear of the interior organs of the person and also problems with digestion.
Here are a number of the conditions and symptoms which will be caused by wearing a slimming belt :

Contraction of the skeletal structure.

Change the situation of body parts.

Heartburn and indigestion.

Fainting thanks to lack of oxygen.

IMPORTANT TIP :

The foremost effective and fastest thanks to reduce and keep your back straight isn't to never wear a weight belt, but to eat a healthy diet and exercise regularly.

Walking, jogging, cycling and swimming are very beneficial exercises for losing weight. Resistance training is additionally beneficial for losing weight and maintaining a healthy body.

You will do twenty minutes of resistance training 3 times every week and do yoga twice every week for the simplest leads to all aspects of your health.

5. STUDY : EATING WHILE WALKING INCREASES WEIGHT

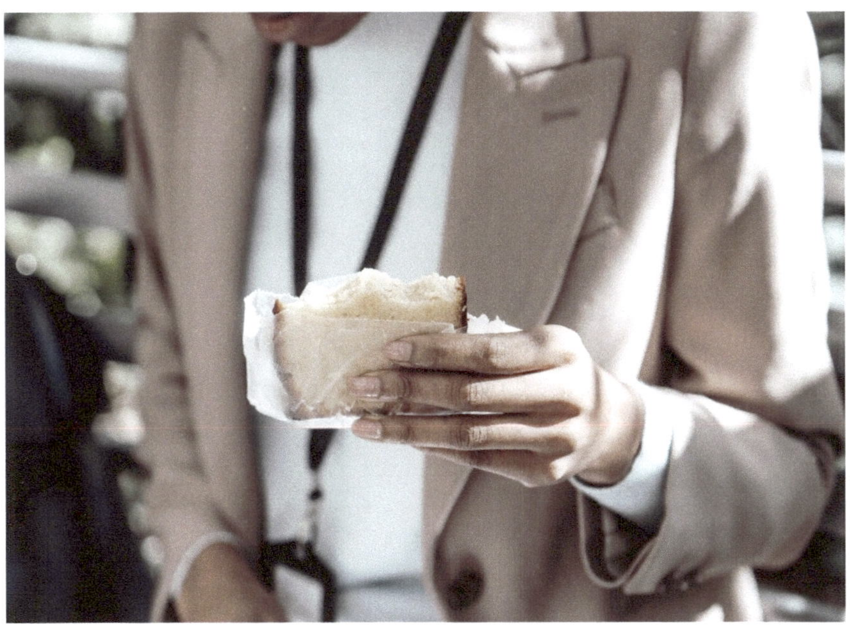

There are many things that we do on a daily basis without feeling like they leave negative effects on our health, so to cope with the hectic and hectic life, most of us tend to eat for the sake of gain, minutes of the day, so what ? is the effect of eating while walking ?

A new British study published in the Journal of Health Psychology has found that anyone who eats on the way to work or any other place without sitting at the table can increase the amount of food they eat during the day and thus gain more. over weight or even become obese.

The researchers, based on the University of Surrey study, indicated that eating food while walking encourages swallowing more than eating it while watching TV or talking with a friend.
The researchers targeted 60 women and they were given breakfast cereal in the form of a cereal bar to be taken in three different cases :

THE FIRST GROUP WAS INVITED TO EAT THIS TABLET WHILE WATCHING TV FOR FIVE MINUTES.

THE SECOND GROUP WAS INVITED TO EAT THEIR FOOD WHILE WALKING.

After this experience, participants filled out forms and underwent a taste test that included four different types of snacks :

CHOCOLATE

CARROTS

GRAPE SEED

POTATO CHIPS.

The amount of this leftover food was measured after the women left, and the researchers found these women's whose dieted and ate a cereal bar for breakfast while walking ate more snacks, especially chocolate.

The study's principal investigator, Professor Jane Ogden, said : "Eating while walking will lead to eating more food later, especially for dieters." On our ability to deal with the effect of eating food on the hunger we feel, or because walking is a type of exercise, which warrants eating larger amounts of food later".

As walking is a type of exercise, it is certainly beneficial, especially for those who want to lose weight, but the timing of walking plays an important role in weight loss or gain.
As this study shows, eating while walking is negative and leads to eating larger amounts of food later in the day and therefore gaining weight, but what about walking after eating ?

A previous study published in 2011 found that walking for half an hour after eating straight is more effective for weight loss than waiting an hour and then walking, as study results indicate that participants lost 1.5 kilograms in a month following the researchers instructions to walk for half an hour after eating immediately.

6. WHAT IS THE DIFFERENCE BETWEEN LOSING WEIGHT AND LOSING FAT ?

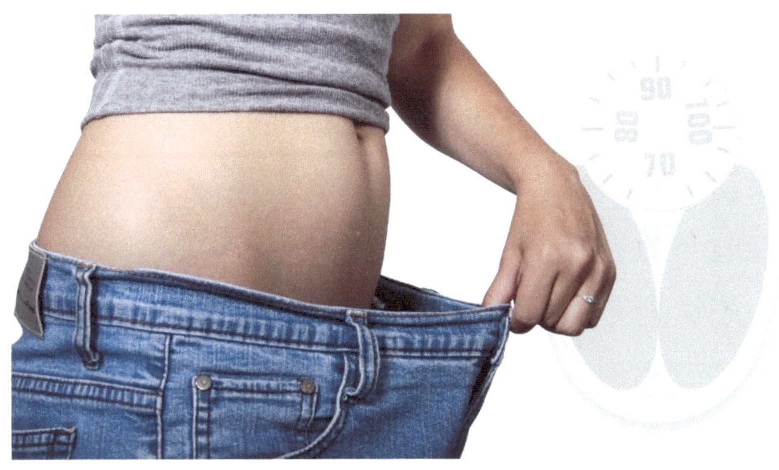

For some people it is confused between losing weight and losing fat, but you need to know the difference if you start to apply the diet to achieve the desired goal.
It is imperative to recognize the difference between these interpretations while dieting in order to achieve the desired result of weight loss.

• MUSCLE LOSS :

Muscles require constant work to maintain them, and some bad practices can lead to loss of muscle, not fat, and then you will notice weight loss, but the body keeps the fat as it is.
Some bad habits lead to loss of muscle, not fat, and these are :

EAT FEWER CALORIES THAN THE BODY NEEDS

Each body needs a specific amount of calories per day, and in the event that this amount is reduced, the burning will not be good.
And if you eat foods that contain fewer calories than the amount appropriate for the body, muscle mass may decrease.

DO NOT EAT FOODS RICH IN PROTEIN

It is not only the amount of food that controls fat burning, but also the quality of the food, as the body needs protein to help muscles grow.
So low protein content in the body will lead to loss of muscle, not fat.

LACK OF EXERCISE

Exercise helps maintain the muscles of the body and also stimulates the burning of accumulated fat.
Therefore, be sure to exercise regularly to lose weight without losing muscle.

• WATER LOSS :

One of the fastest ways to lose weight in a short time is to lose fluids in the body, but this is not an effective method because the weight returns quickly after regaining fluids without getting rid of fat.

This is called a quick diet or a chemical diet for losing weight quickly, which many women resort to before events.

Also, this method of weight loss will affect health, resulting in weakness of muscles and body systems as it does not get the integrated nutrients it needs.

In addition, the lack of water in the body causes an imbalance in metabolism and high sensitivity to insulin.

One of the most important ways to lose water from the body is to give up carbohydrates, despite the importance of eating them in small amounts.

• FAT LOSS :

The main goal of a diet is to lose the most amount of fat, and there is an inverse relationship between fat loss and muscle growth, as well as increased fluidity.

The more the body burns, the better it helps in building muscle and the high fluid content in the body is good for maintaining health.

All methods that help lose fat without losing muscle mass and water should be used, including :

Eat a healthy diet : It is not recommended to eat specific types of food, but rather to eat various foods in small amounts.

And you need to increase the number of vegetables and fruits during the diet, so that the body receives the vitamins and nutrients it needs.

Drink Water : Help to drink water to increase body metabolism and thus increase the burn, so you should drink at least 8 glasses of water per day.

Exercise: Exercise helps burn fat in a large percentage while following the diet.

7. WAYS TO GET RID OF SAGGING SKIN AFTER LOSING WEIGHT

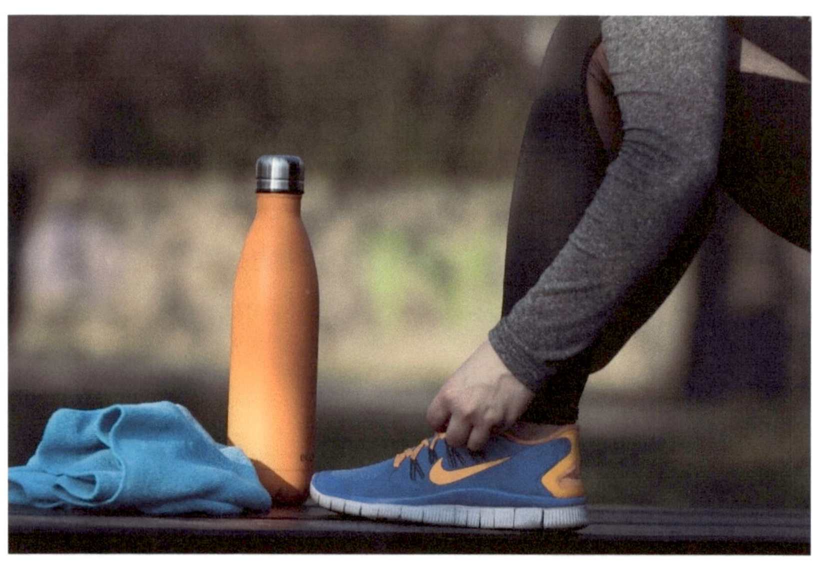

Losing weight causes saggy skin, especially when you're not exercising, and there are ways to reduce sagging skin after losing weight.

After successfully getting rid of excess weight, you will be faced with another problem that you should pay attention to, which is sagging skin, as most people who lose a lot of weight suffer from it, especially in the absence of it exercise.

Hence, there are certain methods that you need to follow that reduce the chances of sagging skin after losing weight.

Factors that increase sagging skin after losing weight.
Certain factors play a major role in increasing sagging skin after weight loss.

• NAMELY AGE :

As age progresses, the skin becomes more elastic, which allows it to sag more.

• GENETIC FACTORS :

Genes affect the tolerance of the skin and the response to any changes.

• HOW MUCH WEIGHT HAS BEEN LOST :

When a large amount of weight is lost in a short period of time, the skin has no chance to shrink, but it continues to stretch and sag later.

• NOT EATING A BALANCED DIET :

Your skin may not be healthy and balanced if you do not eat a healthy and integrated diet during the diet, and thus increase its softness.
Also, not drinking large amounts of water will lead to the same problem as the skin needs hydration to maintain its health.

• LACK OF EXERCISE :

This helps to firm the skin and reduce the possibility of sagging during weight loss.

• LOSE WEIGHT THROUGH SURGERY :

As liposuction surgery results in rapid weight loss, it means sagging skin after the operation.

• HOW TO AVOID SAGGING SKIN AFTER LOSING WEIGHT :

During the period of weight loss, it is recommended to follow these tips to avoid sagging skin later :

SLOW WEIGHT LOSS

This allows the skin to gradually reduce in size along with the weight reduction as it preserves muscle mass while losing fat.
The ideal weight to lose it for the week is 1 to 2 kg at most.

EXERCISE

Exercise helps to tighten the skin and not show sagging, so it is recommended to exercise for the area where the fat is increased.

ADOPT A PROPER DIET

Since losing weight does not mean deprivation and a rigorous diet, it is necessary to eat various foods in appropriate amounts, which ensures the preservation of the health of the skin.

DRINK PLENTY OF WATER

The daily ration of water is not less than 8 glasses per day, it helps moisturize the skin and reduce the risk of sagging.

• WAYS TO GET RID OF SAGGING SKIN AFTER LOSING WEIGHT :

And in the event that sagging skin appears after losing extra weight, this sagging can be reduced in some ways, including :

MAINTAIN SKIN HYDRATION

Drinking large amounts of water helps reduce sagging and moisturizer should be used for the skin.

PROTECT THE SKIN FROM THE SUN

Because the sun contributes to greater sagging, it is recommended that you apply sunscreen and avoid the heat of the sun as much as possible.

EXERCISE TARGETING AREAS OF SAGGING SKIN

This can help restore balance in muscle mass and prevent sagging skin.

STOP SMOKING

This is one of the bad habits that affects the health of the skin and makes it more elastic, and thus increases its softness, and smoking leads to the speed of aging of the skin.

EAT ADEQUATE AMOUNTS OF PROTEIN

There is a close relationship between protein and youthful skin, and therefore it is necessary to eat adequate amounts of protein.

INCREASE THE NUMBER OF VEGETABLES AND FRUITS

The body needs vitamins and minerals to maintain general health and the health of the skin in particular.

WRAP THE SKIN WITH NYLON

A method that helps shrink soft skin, but does not remove it permanently, so some natural oils are applied in addition to petroleum jelly on the sagging area and then wrap it with nylon and stay on for at least two hours before disposing of it.

This is repeated for 10 days in a row for best results.

8. STAPLES AT LUNCH FOR WEIGHT LOSS

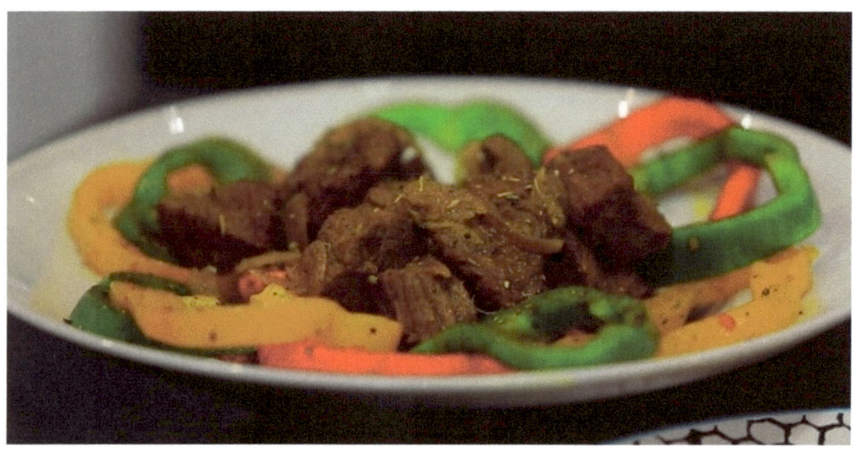

There are certain foods that promote weight loss, especially when eaten for lunch, and therefore it is recommended to include them in the daily diet to increase your burn.

Dieting does not mean starving, as there are many foods that can be eaten while dieting without causing weight gain, but instead can help increase fat burning.

Here is a list of essential breakfast foods to increase burn rates.

• VEGETABLES :

The salad plate is one of the most important lunch meals because it helps to feel full for a long time and thus reduce the consumption of other foods that can lead to weight gain.

It is recommended to add various green vegetables to the salad dish, such as watercress, cucumber, parsley, lettuce and pepper of different colors.

In addition to the salad dish, cooked vegetables should be eaten without adding any oil, ghee, or fat to be healthy and help with weight loss.

Spinach is considered one of the most important leafy vegetables that provide the body with important nutrients such as iron, and it is characterized by its low calorie content.

Broccoli should also be included among the staple foods during the diet as it is low in calories and has many benefits and helps rid the body of toxins.

You can also eat cabbage and Brussels sprouts in this delicious fat-burning vegetable soup.

• FATTY FISH :

Oily fish contain important nutrients for the body, especially omega-3s, which reduces inflammation and thus reduces the risk of obesity.

In addition, oily fish improves thyroid function to produce hormones that promote combustion and maintain metabolism.
Oily fish also make the body feel full without eating a large number of calories.
The fatty fish are mackerel, sardines, salmon and tuna.

• LEAN MEAT :

Fat causes weight gain and many diseases because it causes clogging of the arteries which affects heart health, so you should avoid eating high fat meat.
On the other hand, it is advisable to eat lean meat, as it provides the body with protein which helps reduce the feeling of hunger and increase the levels of burning, and protein can be obtained from meat and chicken.

• BOILED POTATOES :

Although potatoes are a starch that leads to weight gain, they can help to lose it if eaten boiled, as potatoes increase the feeling of fullness for a long time, and therefore it is advisable to eat them a small amount during lunch.

• LEGUMES :

Legumes contain a high percentage of protein and fiber, which are nutrients that help you feel full, so it's best to eat legumes for lunch, like lentils, white beans, and kidney beans.
But at the same time, legumes can cause digestive upset in some people, and therefore overeating is not recommended, and it is better to add cumin to them to reduce bloating and gas.

• SOUP :

Soup should be eaten among the main dishes at lunch, as it helps to feel full more than other foods, as it contains a large percentage of liquids and vegetable soup is one of the best types of soups for losing weight.
But the soup should be free from fat which causes weight gain, and it is better not to add large amounts of salt which hinders weight loss.

• WHOLE GRAINS :

It is not better to eat bread, white rice, or pasta made with white flour for lunch, and it should be replaced with the types made with brown flour, as its calories are lower and therefore will not cause of weight gain like white flour.

9. HOW TO MAINTAIN WEIGHT AFTER DIETING

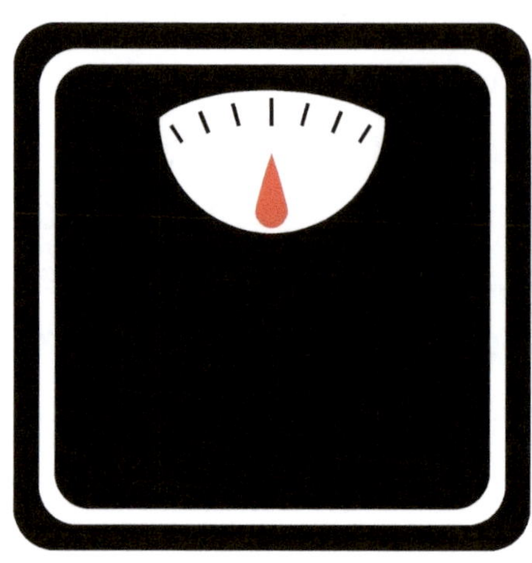

After the stage of weight loss is completed, certain measures need to be taken to ensure that the weight does not come back and to maintain the physical shape of the body throughout life.
One of the big challenges that many people face is losing weight.
During the diet course, many difficulties and obstacles arise to achieve the desired result.
Therefore, methods should be followed to ensure that the ideal weight is maintained after losing many calories, as many studies have shown that a small number of people have the ability to maintain their weight after dieting.

• REASONS TO GAIN WEIGHT AFTER A DIET :

There are some common reasons that lead to regaining weight after losing it, and these are :

Eat unhealthy foods After feeling deprived for a long time, it is difficult to resist many foods that cause weight gain, and over time the weight starts to increase again.

Reduced Burn: This is the result of not following a healthy approach to eating foods, which helps burn fat by eating small meals at varying intervals.

LACK OF EXERCISE

Which helps to burn and not to gain weight, therefore physical activity gradually decreases, which facilitates weight gain, especially with increased food intake.
Methods of maintaining weight after finishing the diet.
To increase the chances of maintaining your weight after following a healthy diet, this step should be well planned by making lifestyle adjustments through certain procedures, including:

COMMITMENT TO EAT BASIC AND SUBSIDIARY MEALS

You should have a breakfast that helps you feel full throughout the day, as well as an increase in energy that helps increase physical activity.
Other meals also contribute to burning, especially small meals, which are vegetables and fruits.
Food should be eaten on time and not late breakfast is no later than nine o'clock, lunch is two to three in the afternoon, and dinner is six to seven in the evening.

REGULAR EXERCISE EVERY DAY

And considering it as an essential part of daily chores, it plays an important role in maintaining weight and not gaining weight later.
Exercise helps burn extra daily calories and increase your metabolism.
It is recommended to practice a brisk walk every day for 30 minutes, as this ensures the stability of the weight.

PAY ATTENTION TO PROTEIN INTAKE

Protein helps reduce appetite and promote a feeling of fullness, and therefore not feel hungry and eat more food, and this is because it increases the levels of certain hormones that stimulate satiety.

In addition, the consumption of protein steadily increases the metabolism and the burning process in the body.

It is recommended to have a variety of protein sources when consuming, and not to limit yourself to just one type, whether animal or vegetable protein.

MEASURE YOUR WEIGHT REGULARLY

Monitoring weight can be an effective way to prevent it from gaining ground, as it serves as a warning tool if you are gaining extra calories to stop bad eating habits.

It is not necessary to take a daily weight measurement, but it can be every three to four days.

LIMIT CARBOHYDRATE INTAKE

Increasing the intake of carbohydrates will again significantly contribute to weight gain, so it is best not to increase them.

It is recommended to replace foods made from white flour with those made from brown flour, as they are much lower in calories.

DO NOT GIVE IN TO WEIGHT GAIN

An important measure that reduces the possibility of gaining weight after losing it is to not give in to eating a lot even after frequently eating large meals.

You need to be careful and stop the mistakes before you reach a stage where it is difficult to control the appetite, because it is okay to enjoy delicious meals for a few days, but it should not be prolonged for a long time.

PREPARATION OF EVENTS AND HOLIDAYS

If you have a special occasion or a vacation when you need to eat different high calorie foods, you should prepare for it by maintaining the weight in the period leading up to these times.

So, when you mess up a healthy diet during this time, there won't be much weight gain.

EAT A FREE MEAL

Even with a healthy diet, it is advisable to have a free meal at the end of the week to help increase your burn and increase your enthusiasm for supplementing the right diet.

But don't go past a meal in which you eat whatever you want from fatty foods and sweets, and get back on track later.

DRINK LOTS OF WATER

There are certain habits that should not be stopped after dieting, the most important of which is drinking water, so do not give up on hydration in your body as it helps to rid it of toxins, increase metabolism. And maintain high combustion levels.

It is recommended to drink 8 cups of water a day, especially in winter when the feeling of thirst is reduced, so do not neglect drinking water.

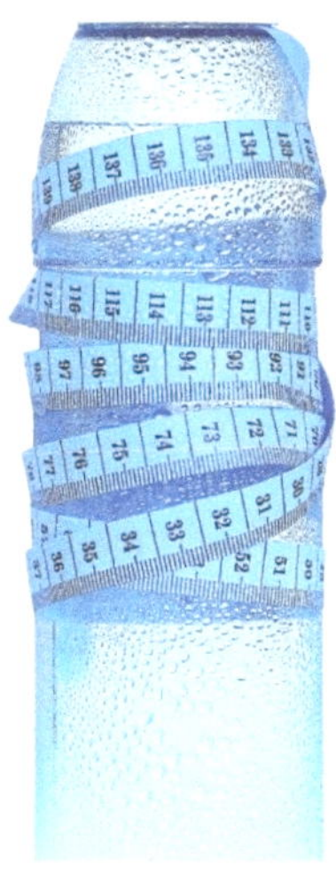

SLEEP WELL

Deprivation of this type is one of the factors that lead to weight gain, as lack of sleep leads to high levels of the hormone ghrelin, known as the hunger hormone because it increases blood pressure. Appetite and, in turn, low levels of the hormone leptin, which is important for controlling appetite.

The less you sleep, the hungrier you will be and the more food you will eat.

Additionally, staying awake late at night increases the chances of eating, which is one of the bad habits that dramatically increases weight.

It is better to sleep no later than ten in the evening and for 7 hours a day.

NOT TO BE SUBJECTED TO STRESSES AND TENSIONS

Stress and anxiety are associated with weight gain as it leads to high levels of cortisol in the body which leads to increased body fat and increased appetite for food.

In addition, stress leads to eating fast, which causes you to eat a lot of food before you feel hungry, but you have to eat slowly.

To reduce stress and stress, there should be a daily plan to perform various tasks and practice relaxation exercises.

OBTAINING EXTERNAL SUPPORT

One of the important things that helps keep the weight off is having people supporting you after you lose the weight because the people around you are more influential, whether they are positive or negative.

When the wife cooks fatty foods, the husband will not be able to resist it, and this applies to all members of the family.

Motivating you to maintain a weight and share a healthy diet will help you maintain your new weight.

EAT MORE HEALTHY FOODS

Since healthy foods are an ideal alternative to harmful foods that lead to weight gain, when you are hungry, you can resort to them to satisfy that desire. Vegetables are at the forefront of these foods and therefore all types of fresh vegetables should be available in the home.

You can also eat many types of fruits that contain vitamins that are important for health and do not cause weight gain, such as apples, guava, and pears.

10. A STUDY SAYS CHEWING GUM SAVES WEIGHT

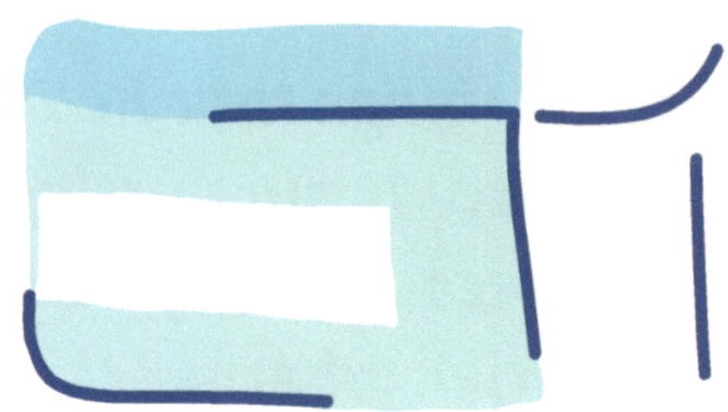

Doctors recommend chewing gum because of its important medical benefit as it increases saliva secretions and cleans teeth of food debris and bacteria stuck there after eating meals, some resort to chewing gum as a solution to lose weight.

DOES CHEWING GUM HELP YOU LOSE WEIGHT ?

A recent scientific study demonstrates the importance of chewing sugar-free gum because the study proved the effectiveness of the gum in controlling appetite and weight management as it is considered the favorite snack of some and people aged 18 to 54 But we use chewing gum as an excuse to lose weight, as we try to overcome the munching "nails" between main meals, especially when we are busy at work, studying, or sitting in front of the TV screen for long periods of time. Long hours, and here we tend to eat large quantities without any monitor

Chewing gum is suitable for work or outside the home, as there is no place to rub the teeth, which contain food residues and bacteria, so the chewing gum helps to clean the teeth from leftover food after meals, because doctors recommend eating sugar-free gum when It has medicinal benefits, as it helps improve the secretion of saliva which contains substances that reduce bacteria, so an "automatic wash" »Oral cavity and teeth cleaning.

And for people who suffer from symptoms of dry mouth, chewing gum is beneficial to them, as the chewing process stimulates the rhythm of salivation, to facilitate and accelerate the feeling of comfort chewing gum removes the face and a feeling of freshness, as well as makes the mouth taste and smell good.

Doctors have advised not to overdo chewing and consuming chewing gum for long periods of time, as this causes increased strain on the chewing muscles and jaw joints, and in exceptional cases, this causes increased strain on the chewing muscles and jaw joints. May cause chewing gum for long periods, the occurrence of damage which is manifested by the appearance of pain in the area of the temples i.e. (above the jaw joints) and the ear and face.

Here are all the methods used in the treatment of obesity!

• DOES CHEWING GUM HELP WITH WEIGHT LOSS ? :

Sugar-free gum, which is only 5-10 calories, can be a healthy alternative to high-calorie "snacks" that are eaten between main meals.

According to the FDA, it has been agreed that chewing sugarless gum is something that helps maintain weight, but obesity can increase the likelihood of developing various diseases such as diabetes, heart disease, and certain types of cancer.

As a result, nutritionists have explained some facts about the importance of chewing gum, including :

Chewing gum has helped reduce hunger after eating a healthy meal, the urge to eat large amounts of food, and the craving for sweets. This fact has been achieved through scientific research published in an American journal called Appetite, and this journal publishes research related to eating behaviors.

Chewing gum burns around 11 calories per hour, but it's not that long. But cutting fewer calories can have a long-term effect, and if you're sitting in front of the TV or the computer, you need to chew gum.

Sugar-free gum is also calorie-free. If used as a substitute for snacks, "nqarish" in this case may aid in weight loss.

TIPS :

In the interest of your health and the health of your body and to preserve your weight, we put in your hands some tips on chewing gum, and what you should do :

After meals, chew a sugar-free gum and avoid snacking on excess "snacks" after meals.

Stress makes you want to eat. So they tried to chew gum in these cases, chewing helps reduce stress and prevent random binge eating.

Chew gum while cooking and preparing meals to avoid distracting certain foods during preparation.

When you go out to eat, chew sugarless gum while you wait for your main course, rather than pieces of bread or other appetizers.

Take sugar-free gum everywhere. Chewing gum is accessible to everyone, delicious, inexpensive, simple and above all, it does not contain calories.

11. BASIC TIPS AND RULES FOR CONTROLLING WEIGHT

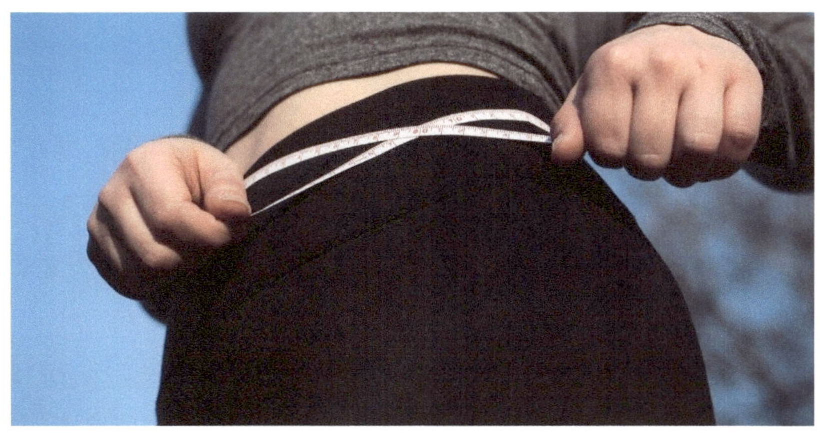

Here are 10 tips and basic rules to help you control your weight and protect yourself from obesity and overweight.

• SUCCESSFUL LIFESTYLE CHANGES FOR WEIGHT LOSS INCLUDE :

COMMITMENT

A person should be enthusiastic about losing weight, because only the patient is able to help himself, but the presence of a doctor or dietitian to set up a special program in addition to family and social support is also important.

THINK POSITIVELY

You shouldn't be thinking about what foods he sacrifices to lose weight, but rather what he gains and benefits from by leaving certain foods.

DEFINITION OF PRIORITIES

Timing is very important, because trying to reduce weight at a time when a person is suffering from other issues will most likely lead to failure. Changing their habits requires great mental and physical effort, so if there are family issues or current issues, the person will not be able to comply with such a difficult decision.

SET A REASONABLE GOAL

Trying to achieve a weight that can be maintained with age and lose weight in a healthy way should be a slow but sustainable process, and a good method is to lose half a kilogram per week for a woman and 1 kilogram for man per week, because the speed of the metabolic system of men is greater, which facilitates weight reduction.

KNOWLEDGE OF HABITS

The person should determine the pattern of eating food and whether he tends to eat when he feels bored, angry, tired, tense or depressed, that is why he should do all work to resist the temptation of food, such as calling a friend for a sports activity or a 30-minute walk, for example.

GRADUAL CHANGE

When determining what behaviors or trends a person wants to change, an important thing to remember is that changes that happen gradually are those that last for a long time.

ADVANCE PLANNING

Old habits can be so ingrained in a person that he practices them without thinking, but mental exercise can help new habits, as if a person imagines himself in a night full of delicious food and suffices with small amounts. Repeating this plan in the mind increases the feeling that it can actually be implemented.

DON'T STARVE

Liquid foods, appetite suppressant pills, and special nutritional formulas are not the solution for long-term excess weight loss, as the daily calorie intake of less than 1200 calories (in women) and under 1400 calories (in men)

Does not ensure adequate nutrition and makes you feel hungry before the date of next meal, and taking appetite suppressant pills is not recommended as its medicinal substance is one of the activity mimics sympathetic nerve that can raise blood pressure contrary to the original goal, and the best way to lose weight is to eat healthier foods and change eating habits, and reducing calories from fatty substances allows a person replacing nutrient-dense foods such as grains, fruits and vegetables.

EXERCISE REGULARLY

Dieting alone can help reduce weight, but if you are accompanied by a brisk walk for half an hour several times a week, it doubles the rate of weight reduction and promotes fat loss and replacement. By muscles, and these changes in the body help to increase the rate of calorie (calorie) burning

KEEP THE SAME PACE OF PROGRESSION

You need to stick to a weight loss program and not let go or go back to your old ways.

THINK ABOUT THE FUTURE

It is not enough to eat and exercise for a few weeks, but rather it is about looking to the future and making these habits part of everyday life.

12. 8 HORMONES THAT CAUSE WEIGHT GAIN IN WOMEN

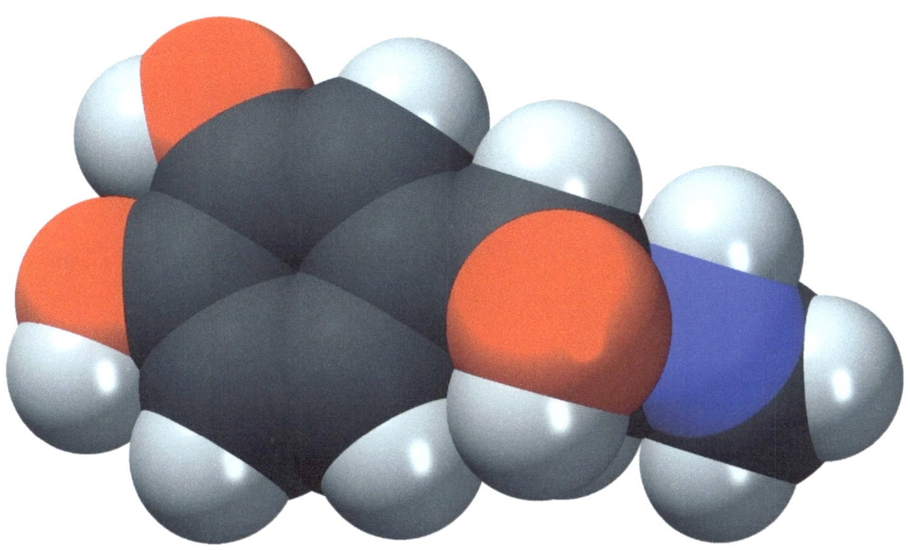

Losing weight is a big challenge for many women, and sometimes hormones are the reason for not losing excess weight. Find out which hormones cause women to gain weight in this article.

Hormones play a role in weight, and its disorder can lead to weight gain in some women, here are the most important hormones that cause weight gain in women as follows :

• HORMONES CAUSE WEIGHT GAIN IN WOMEN :

Below, we review the most important hormones that cause weight gain in women :

THYROID HORMONES

The thyroid gland produces three different types of hormones that regulate metabolism, sleep, heart rate, growth, brain development, and more. Some women develop hypothyroidism, which contributes to weight gain, in addition to certain other symptoms, such as :

Depression.

Constipation.

Tired.

High cholesterol level.

Decreased heart rate.

Also, hypothyroidism causes fluid to build up and retention in the body, causing the body to appear swollen as if it has increased by a few grams.

THE HORMONE INSULIN

The hormone insulin is produced by the pancreas and works to transport glucose to the body's cells to be used for energy or stored as fat, in order to maintain blood sugar levels.
But eating a lot of processed and processed foods, alcohol, sugary drinks, and unhealthy foods can cause what's called insulin resistance.
With insulin resistance, cells are unable to respond to insulin and take advantage of glucose, increasing its accumulation in the blood, leading to high blood sugar, weight gain, and type 2 diabetes.

LEPTIN

In normal cases, the secretion of the hormone leptin indicates a feeling of fullness to stop eating, and it can be among several hormones that cause weight gain in women.
As excessive consumption of high sugar and processed foods leads to supplying your body with high levels of fructose, which turns into stored fat in the liver, abdomen and other areas of the body.

Usually fat cells secrete the hormone leptin, but if you eat foods high in sugar and accumulate more fat in the body, you produce higher amounts of this hormone.

This causes the body to sag and the brain to stop recognizing feelings of fullness, eating more fat, and gaining weight.

GHRELIN

Also called the hunger hormone, it is secreted by the stomach, small intestine, brain, and pancreas, and is one of the many hormones that cause weight gain in women.

As the secretion of high levels of this hormone can lead to weight gain, the hungrier you are, the more you eat.

And a previous scientific study found that the level of this hormone was higher in obese people compared to others.

THE HORMONE CORTISOL

This hormone is secreted by the adrenal gland, especially when a person is feeling nervous, depressed, anxious, and angry, and the role of this hormone lies in each of the following :

Regulating energy in the body : By regulating the way the body uses carbohydrates, proteins and fats for its various tasks.

Boost energy : to even help manage stress and restore balance afterwards.

But the increased secretion of the hormone cortisol causes high blood sugar, which leads to increased insulin secretion in the body and an increase in the amount of accumulated fat and therefore weight gain, which in turn leads to increased insulin secretion in the body is one of the many hormones that cause weight gain in women too.

MELATONIN

Melatonin is secreted by the pineal gland in the body and works to maintain a circadian rhythm. The levels of this hormone increase in the evening until late at night and fall again early in the morning.

When the levels of this hormone increase during sleep, the body temperature drops slightly and the growth hormone is released to help the body repair the damage.

Unfortunately, many of us don't maintain this pace and order, which increases stress and ultimately leads to weight gain.

ESTROGEN HORMONE

Estrogen helps regulate metabolism and body weight, so a decrease in estrogen levels in the premenopausal stage can lead to weight gain, especially in the lower body.

Also, an increase in estrogen levels as a result of eating an estrogen-rich diet or taking certain medications can cause your blood sugar levels to rise and weight gain.

TESTOSTERONE

This hormone helps burn fat, strengthen bones and muscles, and improve sexual desire.

A woman's testosterone is produced in the ovaries, but stress and aging contribute to low levels of the hormone, which is associated with decreased bone and muscle density and a higher risk of obesity.

13. WEIGHT LOSS OILS

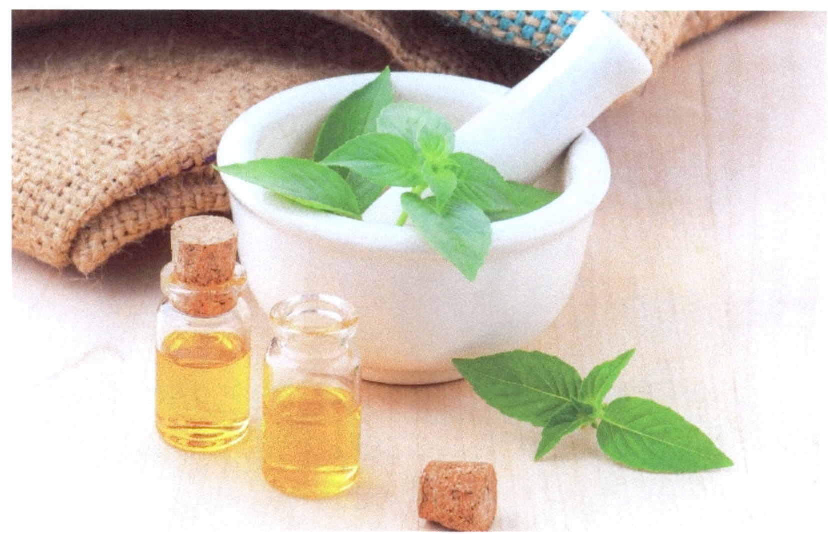

There are many ways to help lose weight and burn fat, and certain types of oils help improve the burning process while on the diet.

Natural oils are used in the treatment of many health conditions, such as dry skin and hair loss, and they can also be used to reduce inflammation, and the benefits of oils are not limited to treating various problems, but they can also contribute to losing excess weight.

Here are the most important natural oils that help with weight loss.

• COCONUT OIL :

Coconut oil increases feelings of fullness and helps regulate appetite, as well as coconut oil reduces inflammation, increases levels of good cholesterol in the blood, and increases insulin sensitivity.
To stimulate fat burning, it is recommended to add a little coconut oil to food daily, or to eat a teaspoon of it.

• LEMON OIL :

Lemons have fat burning properties, and this also applies to lemon oil, which is considered to be one of the best oils for weight loss.
This is because lemon oil helps to flush toxins from the body, thereby stimulating and increasing energy levels, improving fat digestion and stimulating the metabolic process which increases fat burning.
Lemon oil also helps treat arthritis which prevents exercise.

• OLIVE OIL :

Although its calories are not low, olive oil can help with weight loss, as it is one of the healthy fats that lead to feeling full when eating a little, which guarantees not to eat too much.
You can add a spoonful of olive oil to a green salad or roast chicken and meat.

• LAVENDER OIL :

Lavender oil helps to increase the feeling of relaxation, relieve tension and treat sleep disturbances, which are important for increasing fat burning in the body as stress negatively affects hormones and thus hinders the process. burning. Difficulty sleeping at night can lead to weight gain, due to increased secretion of the hunger hormone and consumption of more food, but in the case of inhaling oil of lavender, it will help to fall asleep quickly.

To achieve an effective result, it is recommended to put three drops of lavender oil on the wrists and neck from the back before bedtime.

• GRAPEFRUIT OIL :

Grapefruit oil promotes the breakdown of fat in the body by activating enzymes, and it also contains powerful compounds that support metabolism and cleanse the lymph nodes, allowing them to transport nutrients to the tissues.

To reap the benefits of grapefruit oil, massage the abdomen to help reduce fat, and it can also be used to reduce hunger pangs by adding two drops to a cup of water and drinking it, or by placing two drops on the wrists or chest.

• GINGER OIL :

GINGER OIL HELPS STIMULATE DIGESTION, REDUCE INFLAMMATION, AND REDUCE SUGAR CRAVINGS. GINGER ALSO BURNS FAT AND INCREASES METABOLISM IN THE BODY.
YOU CAN ADD TWO DROPS OF GINGER OIL TO A CUP OF LUKEWARM WATER AND DRINK IT ONCE A DAY, OR ADD A FEW DROPS TO A LUKEWARM WATER BATH AND INHALE IT.

• CINNAMON OIL :

Cinnamon is used to regulate blood sugar and insulin levels, and by balancing blood sugar, cinnamon oil can reduce sugar cravings and overeating, as well as reduce feelings of fatigue and emotional stress.
To use cinnamon oil, add 5 drops of it to a teaspoon of coconut oil and place it on the wrists or abdomen.

• PEPPERMINT OIL :

Peppermint oil has a strong aroma that helps reduce appetite and increase feelings of fullness, and it is recommended to inhale it every two hours to reduce feelings of hunger.

For more benefits, peppermint oil can be mixed with other oils to inhale together, such as grapefruit oil and lemon oil.

14. GENETIC EXAMINATION AND GENETIC MAP TO HELP WITH WEIGHT LOSS

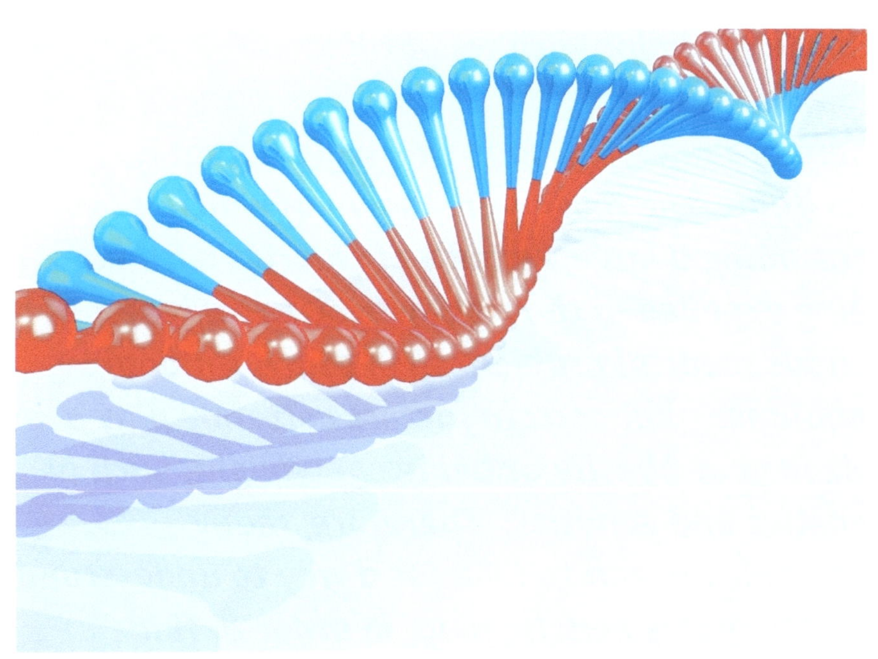

One of the modern trends in medicine that helps you improve your health nutritionally is the nutritional footprint and genetic map. Let us inform you about its relationship in finding solutions for those suffering from overweight as follows :

In a truly unique revolution in the world of medicine, the subject of gene mapping and DNA fingerprint examination has arisen, through which the basic structure of a person's genes is determined to show the relationship between health problems and the risk of infection and the body's interaction with food and various sports. Here we will be dedicated to talking about the relationship between genes and how their knowledge helps with weight loss.

There are many reasons why weight gain is inevitable, the most well-known of which is consuming a large amount of calories without being expelled in the right way. Or as a result of a serious medical problem such as a hormonal imbalance. But certain factors certainly play a role in your obesity or being overweight, such as genetics and genetics. Therefore, many companies began to look for a way to understand and study this genetic map, in order to find solutions that could help with weight loss.

• WHAT IS GENETIC SCREENING ? :

This is an exam done by taking a sample of blood or a swab from inside the patient's mouth to collect DNA. Next, specialist scientists in the lab examine forms of single nucleotides, or polymorphs, because single nucleotide polymorphism is the most common type of genetic variation in people.

According to the Mayo Clinic, the promoting companies are examining weight loss genes by focusing on genes that play a role in weight gain and The exam provides you with information on genes related to metabolism and fat absorption, thereby determining the effect of nutrients on the body and helping to develop a special diet for your condition.

• HOW EFFECTIVE ARE GENETICALLY ENGINEERED DIETS :

Several studies have shown that following a specially designed diet based on the genetic map may actually have a positive effect.

In a study conducted by Stanford University, it was found that participants who followed a genetic-based diet lost about 5.3% of their weight compared to those who followed a diet unrelated to genetics losing about 2% of their weight, 3% of their body weight.

According to the results of the previous study, the results were more striking when following common commercial diets, such as the Atkins diet high in protein and low in carbohydrates, or by following the Ornish diet low in fat. They did not experience any significant results compared to those who followed the genetically linked diet and lost 6.8% of their weight. Compared to the results of the first team, whose members lost only about 1.4% of their body weight.

• IN CONCLUSION :

So, it seems that the results are promising when it comes to genetics and their intervention in the weight loss process, but definitely before taking genetic tests you need to learn the skills of a good lifestyle and how to deal with it.

Your weight through good nutrition and healthy habits every day, and always remember that prevention is better than a pound of treatment.

THANK YOU FOR YOUR PURCHASE

Don't Forget To Let Us A Feedback
To Upgrade This Book.

Follow Our Page For More Books Soon.

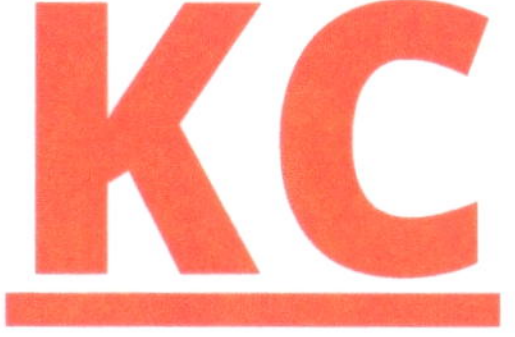

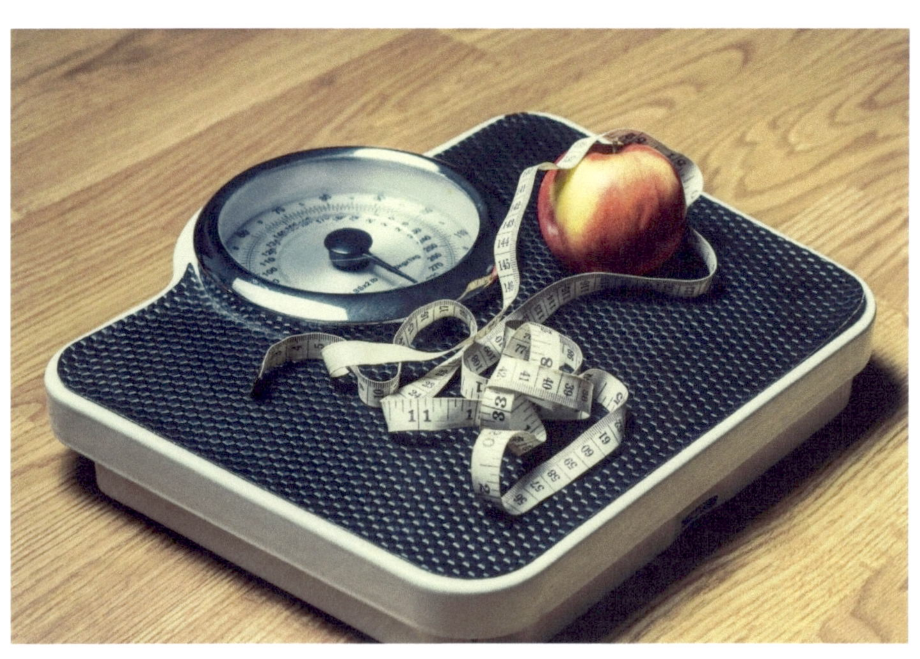

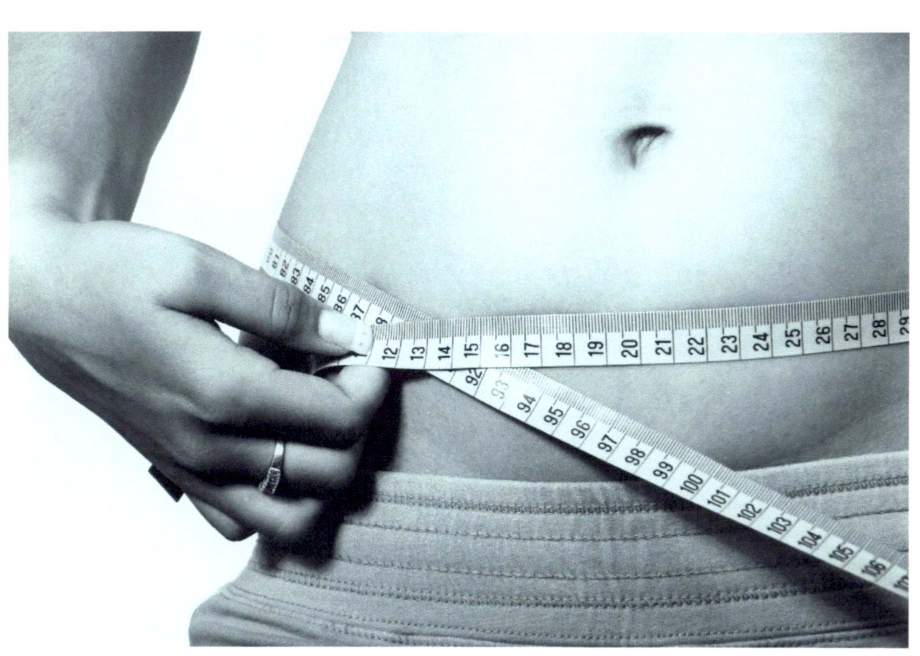

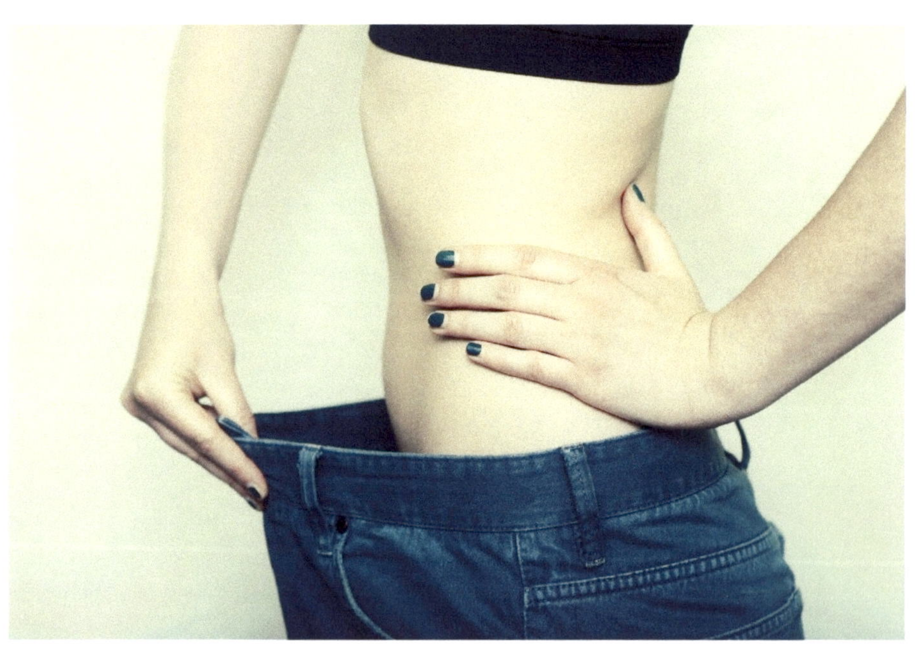

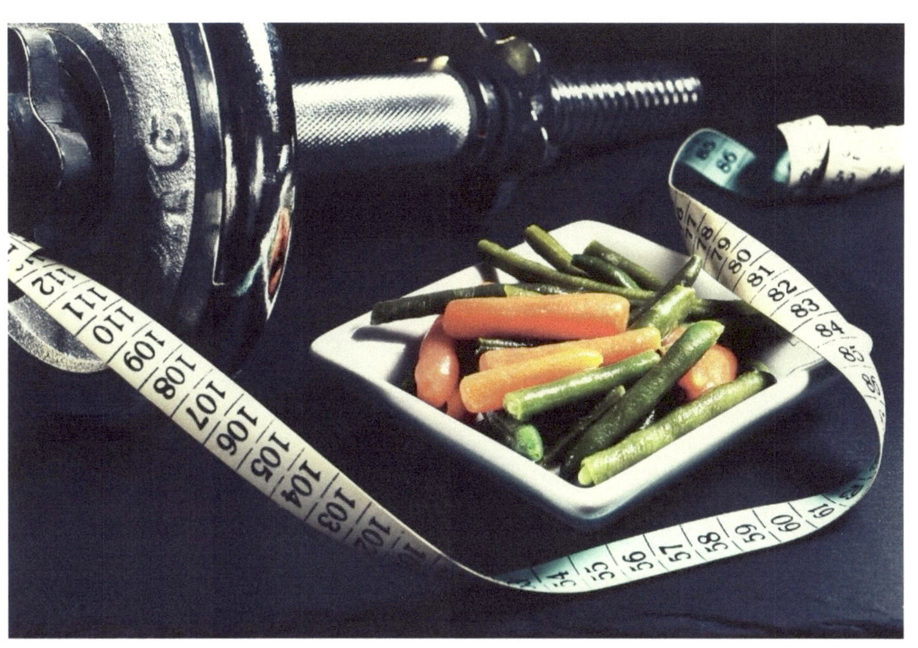

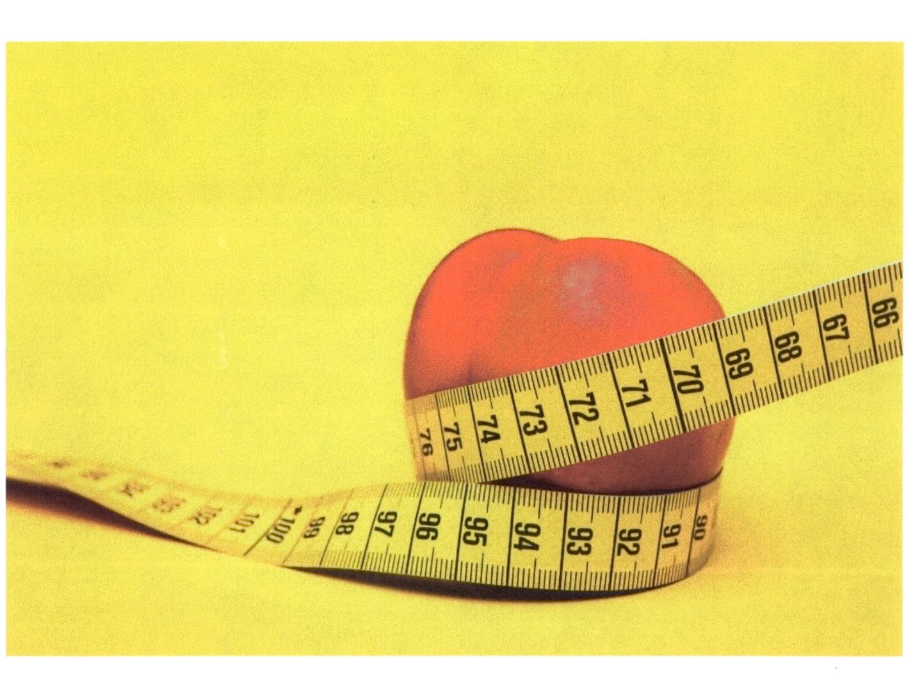

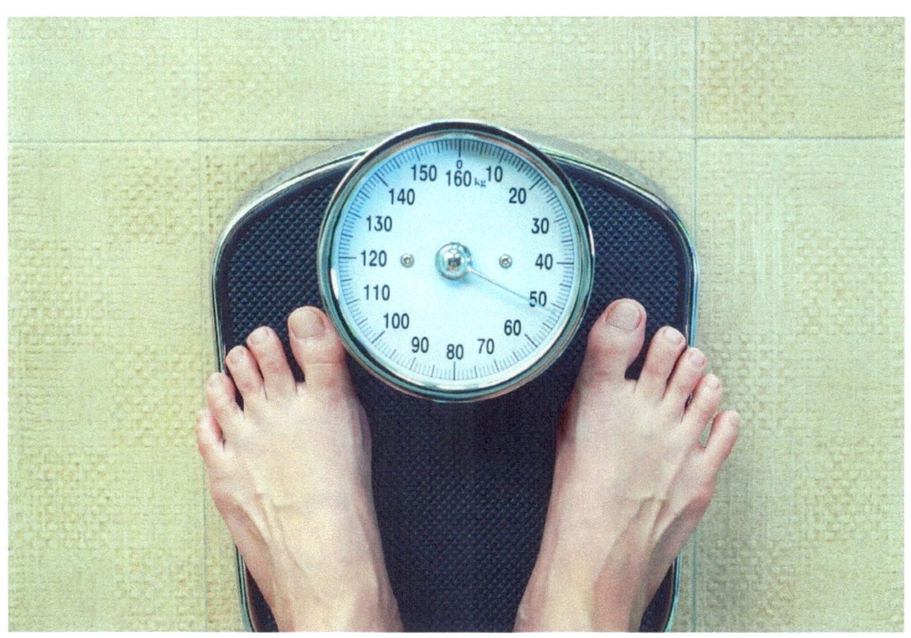

150
140
130
120
110
100
90 80 70
160 kg
0
10
20
30
40
50
60

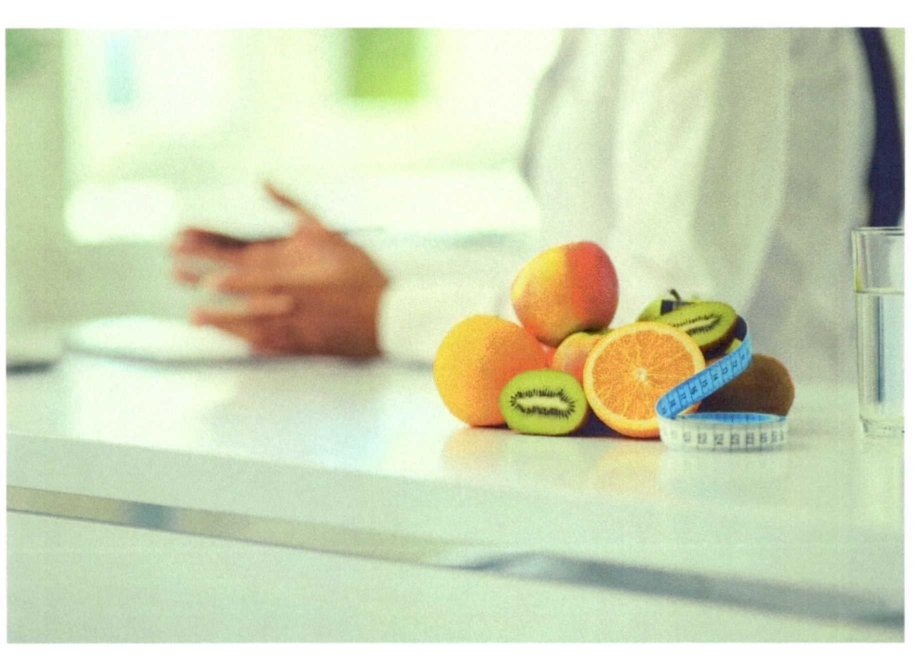

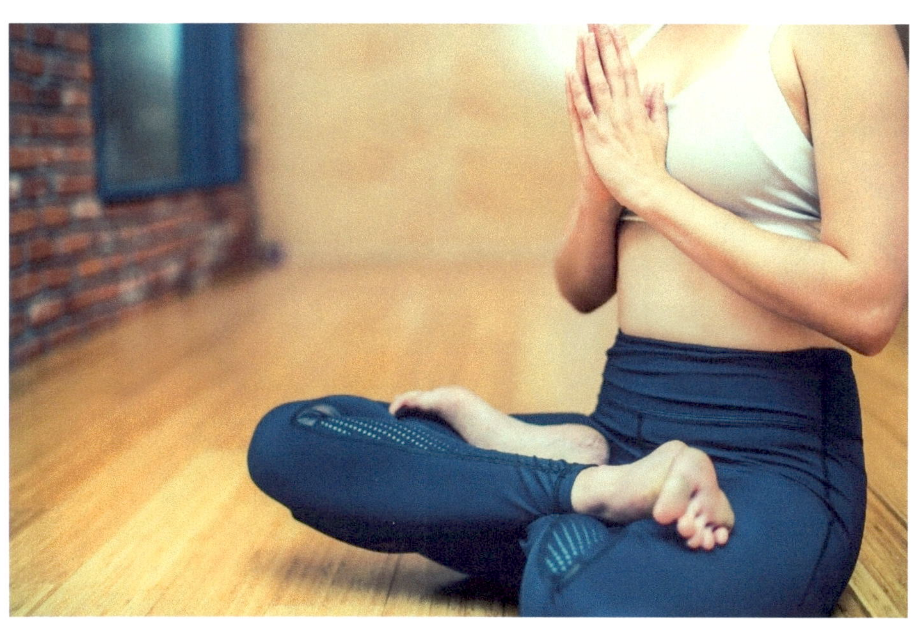

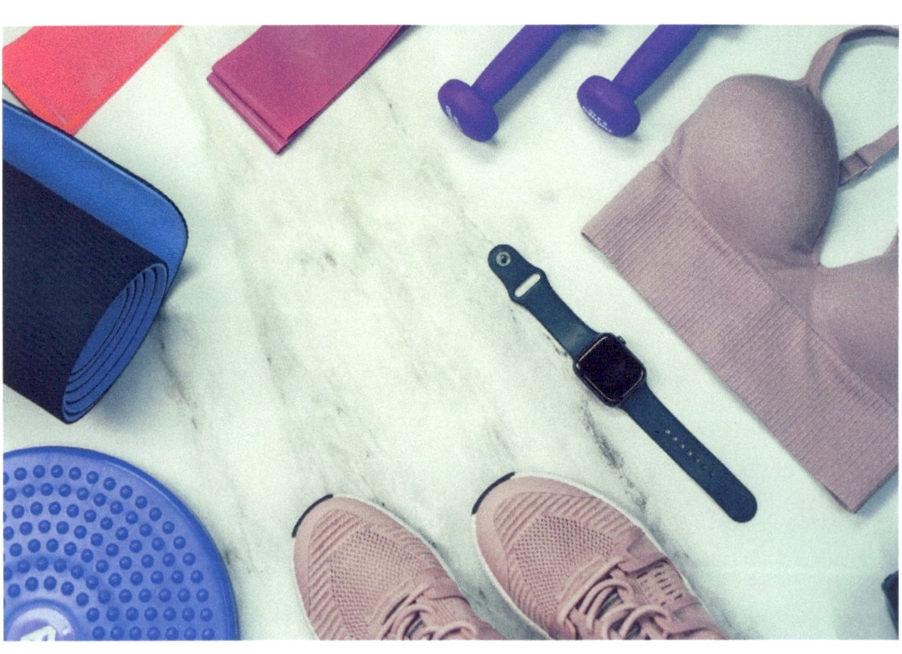